KETO MEAL PREP

—————— ❧❧❧ ——————

Table of Contents

INTRODUCTION

In The United States, the obesity epidemic continues to rise. 38% of our adult population are considered obese. Another 33% of persons are considered overweight. This is according to The Centers For Disease Control and Prevention.

The numbers are even higher for women. Women, because of our child-bearing bodies, have other factors we must contend with. Elevated estrogen levels and different female hormones have our bodies already at a higher fat percentage. Obesity is medically defined as having a body index (BMI) of more than 30%. Personally, I have dieted almost my entire adult life. I'm now over the age of 50. I began to look for a better way to approach fooA Ketogenic is a diet known as a very low carb diet. It is a high fat, moderate protein and low carb intake diet. It turns your body into a fat burning machine. There is a much more scientific explanation but basically you force your body to produce ketones in the liver to be used for energy. On the opposite end, eating foods high in carbs and sugars your body will produce glucose and raise insulin levels.

Although ketogenics is new to many, it was around as early as the 1920s. The keto lifestyle can have a healthful effect on serious health conditions, like cardiovascular diseases and diabetes. It improves levels of HDL cholesterol.

To enter into ketosis, you need to reduce your carbs to under 50 grams a day. Ideally 25-30 carbs max. Your fat intake should be about 75% of your meals and about 15% protein. It varies from person to person, but with consistency you should be able to get into ketosis within 3-14 days.

When you consume a high amount of carbohydrates your metabolism spends most of the time burning carbs for fuel. You never get to burn stored fat. If you decrease the amount of available carbs, your body must switch to burning your fat.

CHAPTER ONE
THE BASIC PRINCIPLES OF THE KETOGENIC DIET

The ketogenic diet is a diet based on a process called ketosis. It is a specific state of the body, which is characterized by an elevated level of ketones in the blood, which occurs due to the conversion of fats into fatty acids and ketones. This occurs when the body gets only very small amounts of carbohydrates over a certain period of time. When you start with this type of diet, your body goes through several changes. 24-48 hours after the beginning of this diet, the body starts to use ketones in order to use the energy stored in fat cells more efficiently. In other words, the primary source of energy becomes fat (fatty acids), instead of carbohydrates (glucose). Because of that, during ketosis it is not a problem to eat food with higher amounts of fat, than would otherwise seem reasonable. This way the body is rapidly losing weight (specifically fat). In addition, the loss of muscle tissue (proteins) is minimal, since the vast majority of food consumed during ketosis, also contains relatively large amounts of proteins that are good for your muscles.

Although ketosis is the basis of the ketogenic type of diet, in its strictest form it doesn't need to be kept for long. The state of ketosis can be held up until the body weight is just a few pounds higher than the one that is desired. Then foods with higher amounts of carbohydrates are gradually introduced (rice, beans). In this period, it would be very useful to keep a food intake diary in which daily amounts of taken carbs would be noted. That way you can find the maximum amount of daily carbs that still allow you not to gain weight. Once you discover this parameter, you will no longer have weight-related problems, because you will certainly learn to take account of the calories and amounts of carbs, proteins and fats that you consume daily. That way you will get to know your body better, in terms of the maximum "allowable" daily intake. Because of that, we could say that the ketogenic diet is, in a way, a procedure for learning habits that will ensure that you never return to the old potentially problematic overweight levels.

There are many types of ketogenic diets , but they all have in common one basic principle: the intake of high amounts of proteins and fats, and minimal amounts of carbohydrates. Which exact diet you will choose isn't as important, as long as it will allow you to enter ketosis, which is the basis of the biological mechanism that will help you lose weight efficiently.

Low carb diets have advantages and disadvatages.

The reason low carb has a bad rap is that people say they are low carb, but really aren't. It's like saying you're low calorie while eating a bowl of ice cream with a donut on top. The people who give low carb a bad name do not follow the basic principle of low carb: a constant, steady stream of carbs that have a total during the day of less than a set amount, usually 100g, and all of the carbs come from fruits and vegetables. Of course, some diets are more strict and I myself keep to below 70g per day.

So, who are these people who say they are low carb, but really aren't? Well, they starve themselves of carbs, focus on meats and fats only and then pig out on sugar on the weekends. Then they start all over again. These people are cranky, depressed and miserable. Plus, they aren't losing a pound. They blame the diet and not the dieter who isn't doing it right.

Doctors hate the low carb diet because of these people. You see, when you starve yourself of something, then pig out, you force your body to shift it's metabolism from ketogenic (protein) metabolism to carbohydrate metabolism quickly, and it doesn't like it. It leads to a stressed liver, heart and brain. It produces lots of cortisol, which causes us to hold onto fat and store even more. It layers plaque in our arteries to help reduce the stress. It harms the kidneys because of the toxic burden of switching back and forth.

The focus on meats and fats deprives the body of vital nutrients and the organs start to break down. This kind of dieting makes people sick. This is where many of the myths of the low carb diet come from: these people who are not doing low carb at all.

For those who want to do it right, it requires discipline. It requires long periods of constant, steady streams of carbs, without spikes or indulgences. In fact, it is one of the healthiest diets to be on. Lower carb is the basis of all healthy diets: Mediterranean, vegetarian, diabetic, Atkins and all the others.

BASIC PRINCIPLES OF THE KETOGENIC DIET

Doing it right goes like this:

> Set your carbs: I recommend no less than 60g/day unless under the care of a nutritionist.

> Plan your day around your fruits and vegetables: I recommend no less than 5 servings per day

> Make sure those fruits and vegetables are within your carb counts.

> Flavor with herbs and spices – as many as possible (they have 0 carbs!)

> Fill in with local, organic or natural meats and healthy fats.

Planning this way will allow you to consume many foods, enough to keep you full and happy and provide all the nutrition you require.

There is only one problem with eating low carb the right way. Fruits and vegetables do not have convenient packages to know exactly how many carbs are in them. A pepper is usually about 6g per serving, but can be as low as 4g in the spring to nearly 10g in the fall. But that's OK, you don't need to be that precise, so long as fruits and vegetables make up the biggest part of your diet.

CHAPTER TWO
WHY KETO MEALS

Keto diets have really caught on in the past year and a half and for good reason. It's a great way to not only shed those unwanted pounds quickly, but also a great way to get healthy and stay that way. For those that have tried the Keto Diet and are still on it, it's more than just a diet. It's a way of life, a completely new lifestyle. But like any major shift in our lives it is not an easy one, and it takes an incredible amount of commitment and determination.

Good for some but not for all? Although a ketogenic diet has been used to greatly improve people's quality of life, there are some out there who do not share the majority's way of thinking. But why is that exactly? Ever since we can remember we have been taught that the only way to get rid of the extra weight was to quit eating the fat-filled foods that we are so accustomed to eating every day. So instructing people to eat healthy fats (the key word is healthy), you can certainly understand why some people would be skeptical as to how and why you would eat more fat to achieve weight loss and achieve it fast. This concept goes against everything we have ever known about weight loss.

How Keto Started. Discovered by endocrinologist Rollin Woodyatt in 1921 when he found that 3 water-soluble compounds named aceture, B-hydroxybutyrate and acetoacetate (known together as ketone bodies) were produced by the liver as a result of starvation or if the person followed a diet rich with high fat and very low carbs. Later on that year a man from the Mayo Clinic by the name of Russel Wilder named it the "Ketogenic Diet" and used it to treat epilepsy in young children with great success. But because of advancements in medicine it was replaced.

What Does A Ketogenic Diet Look Like? When the average person eats a meal rich in carbs, their body takes those carbs and converts them into glucose for fuel. Glucose is the body's main source of fuel when carbs are present in the body; on a keto diet there are very low if any carbs consumed which forces the body to utilize other forms of energy to keep the body functioning properly. This is where healthy fats come into play; with the absence of carbs the liver takes fatty acids in the body and converts them into ketone bodies.

An ideal keto diet should consist of:

- 70-80% Fat

- 20-25% Protein

- 5-10% Carbs

You should not be eating more than 20g of carbs per day to maintain the typical Ketogenic diet. I personally ate less than 10g per day for a more drastic experience but I achieved my initial goals and then some. I lost 28 lbs in a little under 3 weeks.

What Is Ketosis? When the body is fueled completely by fat it enters a state called "ketosis" which is a natural state for the body. After all of the sugars and unhealthy fats have been removed from the body during the first couple of weeks, the body is now free to run on healthy fats. Ketosis has many potential benefits related to rapid weight loss, health or performance. In certain situations like type 1 diabetes excessive ketosis can become extremely dangerous, whereas in certain cases paired with intermittent fasting it can be extremely beneficial for people suffering from type 2 diabetes. Substantial work is being conducted on this topic by Dr. Jason Fung M.D. (Nephrologist) of the Intensive Dietary Management Program.

What I Can and Can't Eat. For someone new to keto it can be very challenging to stick to a low-carb diet, even though fat is the cornerstone of this diet you should not be eating any and all kinds of fat. Healthy fats are essential, but what is healthy fat you might ask. Healthy fats would consist of grass-fed meats, (lamb, beef, goat, venison), wild caught fish and seafood, pastured pork & poultrys. Eggs and salt free butters can also be ingested. Be sure to stay away from starchy vegetables, fruit, and grains. Processed foods are in no way accepted in any shape or form on the ketogenic diet. Artificial sweeteners and milk can also pose a serious issue.

Reasons to Avoid Low Carb Diets

Low carb (carbohydrate), high protein diets are the latest dieting craze. However, before you jump on the band wagon, you may want to consider a few things:

1. Low carb (ketogenic) diets deplete the healthy glycogen (the storage form of glucose) stores in your muscles and liver. When you deplete glycogen stores, you also dehydrate, often causing the scale to drop significantly in the first week or two of the diet. This is usually interpreted as fat loss when it's actually mostly from dehydration and muscle loss. By the way, this is one of the reasons that low carb diets are so popular at the moment – there is a quick initial but deceptive drop in scale weight.

    Glycogenesis (formation of glycogen) occurs in the liver and muscles when adequate quantities of carbohydrates are consumed – very little of this happens on a low carb diet.

    Glycogenolysis (breakdown of glycogen) occurs when glycogen is broken down to form glucose for use as fuel.

2. Depletion of muscle glycogen causes you to fatigue easily, and makes exercise and movement uncomfortable. Research indicates that muscle fatigue increases in almost direct proportion to the rate of depletion of muscle glycogen. Bottom line is that you don't feel

energetic and you exercise and move less (often without realizing it) which is not good for caloric expenditure and basal metabolic rate (metabolism).

3. Depletion of muscle glycogen leads to muscle atrophy (loss of muscle). This happens because muscle glycogen (broken down to glucose) is the fuel of choice for the muscle during movement. There is always a fuel mix, but without muscle glycogen, the muscle fibers that contract, even at rest to maintain muscle tone, contract less when glycogen is not immediately available in the muscle. Depletion of muscle glycogen also causes you to exercise and move less than normal which leads to muscle loss and the inability to maintain adequate muscle tone.

   Also, in the absence of adequate carbohydrate for fuel, the body initially uses protein (muscle) and fat. The initial phase of muscle depletion is rapid, caused by the use of easily accessed muscle protein for direct metabolism or for conversion to glucose (gluconeogenesis) for fuel. Eating excess protein does not prevent this because there is a caloric deficit.

When insulin levels are chronically too low as they may be in very low carb diets, catabolism (breakdown) of muscle protein increases, and protein synthesis stops.

4. Loss of muscle causes a decrease in your basal metabolic rate (metabolism). Metabolism happens in the muscle. Less muscle and muscle tone means a slower metabolism which means fewer calories burned 24 hours-a-day.

5. Your muscles and skin lack tone and are saggy. Saggy muscles don't look good, cause saggy skin, and cause you to lose a healthy, vibrant look (even if you've also lost fat).

6. Some proponents of low carb diets recommend avoiding carbohydrates such as bread, pasta, potatoes, carrots, etc. because of they are high on the glycemic index, causing a sharp rise in insulin. Certain carbohydrates have always been, and will always be the bad guys: candy, cookies, baked goods with added sugar, sugared drinks, processed/refined white breads, pastas, and rice, and any foods with added sugar.

These are not good for health or weight loss.

However, carbohydrates such as fruits, vegetables, legumes, whole grain breads and pastas, and brown rice are good for health and weight loss. Just like with proteins and fats, these carbohydrates should be eaten in moderation. Large volumes of any proteins, fats or carbohydrates are not conducive to weight loss and health.

The effect of high glycemic foods is often exaggerated. It does matter, but to a smaller degree than is often portrayed. Also, the total glycemic effect of foods is influenced by the quantity of that food that you eat at a sitting. Smaller meals have a lower overall glycemic effect. Also, we usually eat several types of food at the same time, thereby reducing the average glycemic index of the meal, if higher glycemic foods are eaten.

Also, glycemic index values can be misleading because they are based on a standard 50 grams of carbohydrate consumed.

It wouldn't take much candy bar to get that, but it would take four cups of carrots. Do you usually eat four cups of carrots at a meal?

Regular exercisers and active people also are less effected by higher glycemic foods because much of the carbohydrate comsumed is immediately used to replenish glycogen stores in the liver and muscle.

By the way, if you're interested in lowering insulin levels, there is a great way to do that — exercise and activity.

7. Much of the weight loss on a low carb, high protein diet, especially in the first few weeks, is actually because of dehydration and muscle loss.

8. The percentage of people that re-gain the weight they've lost with most methods of weight loss is high, but it's even higher with low carb, high protein diets. This is primarily due to three factors:

A. You have lost muscle. With that comes a slower metabolism which means fewer calories are burned 24 hours-a-day. A loss of muscle during the process of losing weight is almost a guarantee for re-gaining the lost weight, and more.

B.   You re-gain the healthy fluid lost because of glycogen depletion.

C.   It's difficult to maintain that type of diet long-term.

D.   You have not made a change to a long-term healthy lifestyle.

9.   Eating too much fat is just not healthy. I know you've heard of people whose blood levels of cholesterol and triglycerides have decreased while on a low carb, high protein diet. This often happens with weight loss, but it doesn't continue when you're on a diet high in fat.

There are literally reams of research over decades that clearly indicates that an increase in consumption of animal products and/or saturated fat leads to increased incidences of heart disease, strokes, gallstones, kidney stones, arthritic symptoms, certain cancers, etc. For example, in comparing countries with varying levels of meat consumption, there is a direct relationship between the volume of meat consumption in a country and the incidence of digestive cancers (stomach, intestines, rectal, etc.).

Fat is certainly necessary, and desirable in your diet, but you should eat mostly healthy fats and in moderation.

Manufactured/synthetic "low fat" foods with lots of added sugar are not the answer. Neither are manufactured/synthetic "low carb" foods with artificial sweeteners or added fat. By the way, use of artificial sweeteners has never been shown to aid in weight loss and they may pose health problems.

10. As someone recently told me, "it must work, people are losing weight". People that are truly losing fat on low carb, high protein diets, are doing so because they are eating fewer calories – that's the bottom line. There is no magic – the same can be done on a healthy diet.

11. Low carb diets are lacking in fiber. Every plant-based food has some fiber. All animal products have no fiber. A lack of fiber increases your risk for cancers of the digestive tract (because transit time is lengthened) and cardiovascular disease (because of fiber's effect on fat and cholesterol). It also puts you at a higher risk for constipation and other bowel disorders.

12. Low carb diets lack sufficient quantities of the the   many nutrients/phytonutrients/antioxidants found in fruits, vegetables, legumes, and whole grains, necessary for health and aiding in the prevention of cancer and heart disease. In fact, you need these nutrients even more so when you're consuming too much fat as is often the case on a low carb, high protein diet.

13. Amercans already consume more than twice the amount of protein needed. Add to that a high protein diet and you have far too much protein consumption. By the way, most people don't realize that all fruits, all vegetables, all whole grains, and all legumes also contain protein. Animal products contain larger

quantities of protein, but that may not be a good thing.

Excess dietary protein puts you at a higher risk for many health problems: gout (painful joints from high purine foods which are usually high protein foods), kidney disease, kidney stones, osteoporosis (excess dietary protein causes leeching of calcium from the bones). By the way, countries with lower, healthier intakes of protein also have a decreased incidence of osteoporosis.

14. Low carb, high protein diets cause an unhealthy physiological state called ketosis, a type of metabolic acidosis. You may have heard the phrase, "fat burns in the flame of carbohydrate". Excess acetyl CoA cannot enter the Krebs Cycle (you remember the old Krebs Cycle) due to insufficient OAA. In other words, for fat to burn efficiently and without production of excess toxic ketones, sufficient carbohydrate must be available. Ketosis can lead to many health problems and can be very serious at it's extreme.

15. Bad breath. Often called "keto breath" or "acetone breath", it's caused by the production

of acetones in a state of ketosis. So why the low carb, high protein craze? I believe there are several reasons.

A. Weight loss (mostly muscle and muscle fluid) is often rapid during the first few weeks. This causes people to think they're losing fat rapidly.

B. It gives you "permission" to eat the "bad foods": bacon, eggs, burgers, steak, cheese, etc. and lots of fat.

CHAPTER THREE
HOW TO AVOID COMMMON MISTAKES FOR BEGINNERS

Considering the variety of low carb diet variations out there, it can be hard to decide which one to stick to. For the most part, the low carb approach is perfect if you require to lose 30lbs or more. The most basic low carb diet that seems to work most effectively for individuals works as follows: for nine days you limit your carbohydrate intake to 30 grams everyday. On the 10th day, during the night time, you're allowed a high carbohydrate splurge, but you don't start consuming carbs until after 4pm. After this 10 day period your carb nights are spread out roughly once per week.

It sounds uncomplicated, doesn't it? If you've done any dieting in the past you've quite possibly tinkered around with diets similar to this. However, there are several common pitfalls that either impede progress or cause some people to make hardly any progress. I'll list a couple of them and give some remedies for how to prevent yourself from falling into these traps.

It is very effortless to ingest way too many carbs mainly because of the places you purchase meals. These days a lot of people don't cook and prepare their meals. Many individuals dine out, and although you have a "low carb salad" you will probably find yourself going over your limit by having food that has too many carbs without realizing it. A number of the low fat dressings have approximately 7-10g of carbs, and from time to time when you order a salad they will put greater than three portions. A good practice that my clients use is as simple as just getting the restaurant to put the dressing on the side and all you have to do is separate out a serving.

Going overboard on dairy is yet another frequent blunder. Unless you have a history of enduring dairy well, I strongly recommend most clients to refrain from it entirely when starting off. For most people, dairy can supercharge your urge for food which will cause you to consume too much.

Overeating is the next obvious pitfall. Unless you're eating a lot of whole foods and foods that have marginal processing, it may be easy to overeat. To guarantee your results, its best that you be wary of how much you consume. This is especially true if you're having difficulty experiencing fast enough results. Many of the processed "low carb" foods are very tasty which will either cause you to overeat that food, or just heighten your desire for food for the day which may lead to overeating.

Not receiving a good mix of fat and protein can lead to headaches or the dreaded "ketogenic flu" or keto flu. The signs are a bad throbbing headache and lots of fatigue. This develops as your body adjusts to not having enough carbs using fat instead. When your fat intake is lacking your body may have challenges getting sufficient energy. Don't be afraid of fat, just ensure to keep your saturated fat in check. Sources like avocados, olive oil and coconut oil are fantastic sources. Nuts are okay, you just have to look at the amount of carbs depending on the types of nuts or seeds you take in.

You may still have your steak and various fatty cuts of animal meat. Just make certain that fat sources vary. Coconut oil is a fat that consists of MCTs which your system is able to digest quickly to be used as energy. Other fats take longer to break down and by the time you get that keto flu headache, it can be far too late before symptoms are taken care of.

30 DAYS LOW CALORIES DIET PLAN

A 30 Day Diet Plan is most suitable for people that want to lose weight in a short period. There are several good diet plans available. A detox plan is a good example. A seven day detox meal plan is probably the best choice to lose the most weight in a week. It is a good way to cleanse the body of harmful toxins and lose weight at the same time.

Obviously the main concept of this plan is to consume very little calories. For this meal plan to be successful all of the calories must be counted before being consumed, and a person needs to figure out how many calories they should consume in a day to loose the amount of weight they want. This is calculated by height, weight, gender, age, and body mass index.

This meal plan falls under the category of detox diets. Although the name suggests that any amount of any kind of food can be eaten, in actuality only certain foods are allowed on certain days. The foods allowed to be consumed are vegetables, fruits, lean meat, and skim milk. It is important to drink a lot of water (8 glasses per day).

The Cabbage Soup Diet is another example of a diet plan. It is also considered to be a detox diet.

This meal plan consists of very little fat, all of the cabbage soup a person wants to eat, fruits, vegetables, and lean meat. Cabbage is a negative energy vegetable, this means the body burns more calories eating and digesting it than the cabbage contains. Therefore the more cabbage that is eaten the more weight a person will lose.

The recipe to make the cabbage soup is very simple:

1 small cabbage,
6 medium onions,
7 tomatoes,
2 green peppers.

Chop all the vegetables into small pieces, add water and boil until the vegetables are soft (about 20 minutes) then add salt and spices. On the first day of the diet people can eat all of the fruits except for bananas along with as much cabbage soup as they want.

Day 2. Soup and vegetables and a little bit of boiled potatoes are allowed. The vegetables can be fresh, boiled, or steamed.

Day 3 - Soup, fruit, and vegetables, but no potatoes.

Day 4 - A glass of fat free milk, 2 bananas, fruits, vegetables, and the cabbage soup.

Day 5 - 500 grams of boiled beef or skinless chicken or fish, soup, and tomatoes.

Day 6 - Green vegetables such as lettuce, meat, and of course cabbage soup.

Day 7 - Brown rice, vegetables, fruit juice (sugar free) and soup.

Repeat this for 31 days and you will see great changes.

BELOW SEE 10 HELPFUL HINTS.

1. Eat grains such as high fiber cereal, oatmeal, grits, etc. It is important to have a high fiber diet to keep the body cleansing regularly. Also, these carbohydrates start up your calorie burning machine. This is why fiber cereals are

recommended for breakfast in most healthy eating plans.

2. Eat dark green leafy vegetables daily; such as; spinach, romaine lettuce, dark cabbage, kale and other greens. Dark vegetables are high in fiber and have many nutrients and vitamins that are needed for the body to function at a healthy level, and they are low in calories. Because dark vegetables consist of a large percent of water you can indulge and still lose weight.

3. Eat at least 4 times each day, five when trying to lose weight. By eating often you won't have the opportunity to get hungry and overeat. Secondly, smaller meals are easier for the body to digest, burn off fat and unwanted calories. Because of how our bodies are designed, if you do not feed your body it will go into survival mode and hang onto extra weight versus releasing it.

4. Use portion control to lose weight. Never overeat. Put the appropriate portion of food on your plate. You have to know your portions, for example; steak or chicken should only be 4-5oz; most cooked carbs only 1/2 cup; fresh green

vegetables, because they consist of a high percent of water, you can have 1 cup or more.

5. Read labels. They contain valuable information, such as: how many grams of sugar, sodium, carbs, calories, how much equals 1 serving, etc. Labels are your best friend. If you don't understand them it will be hard to lose weight.

6. Eat breakfast everyday. Breakfast is the most important meal of the day. When a healthy breakfast is eaten it begins the calorie burning machine for the day. Whole grains and oatmeal are highly recommended because they get the metabolism working.

7. Eat fresh fruit but be selective on fruits eaten. Some fruits such as ripe bananas are extremely high in sugar and may be a detriment to your goals, but fruits like blueberries have antioxidants and help build your immune system and are low in calories.

8. Write down everything eaten in a journal. It is important to record everything that you eat. It allows you to see exactly what you are putting in your mouth all day long. It gives you better

insight on why you may not be losing weight. You must record everything that you eat, what time and how much eaten.

9. Don't snack while watching TV. When you eat in front of the TV there may be very little connection on how much your mouth is taking in. This leads to overeating.

10. Don't eat empty calories. If you want to lose weight, make every calorie count. Some foods have great value, while others taste good but have no nutritional value and lots of calories. Know the difference

Balanced Three-Meal Two-Snack Plan

This meal plan is based on splitting daily calorie intake in three meals and two snacks. Mainly, lots of lean protein and veggies are loaded in this diet program.

Breakfast: For starting the day, half cup of egg whites, 1 apple, whole wheat toast and a tablespoon of butter or 2 tablespoons of peanut butter is enough.

Snack: For midday munching, 8 oz. of zero fat Greek yogurt, half cup of berries, 1 tablespoon of agave nectar or a protein bar (200 calories) are considered best.

Lunch: Lunch can include salad made with 3 cups spinach, 2 tablespoons full fat dressing and 4 oz. grilled chicken, along with a half cup garbanzo beans.

Dinner: For ending the day well, you can go for a baked salmon, half sweet potato, and 4 cups roasted vegetables cooked in 2 tablespoons olive oil.

The Vegan Plan

It is one of the latest diet plans, which is mainly popularized by a good number of celebrities. This diet program mainly involves cutting down the intake of processed foods to lose more weight. This plan does not obligate the dieters to stay hungry by cutting down the consumption. It simply replaces the processed food items with healthy ones.

Breakfast: One cup tofu (scrambled), two whole wheat bread slices, two wedges raw cantaloupe and one tablespoon of vegan margarine spread can start the day well.

Snack: One table spoon flax seed in 4 oz. vanilla soy yogurt can serve the purpose.

Lunch: A perfect midday meal includes black bean and sweet potato salad with 2 oz. tofu for a protein kick.

Dinner: One cup quinoa (well cooked) and a single serving of grilled vegetables is suitable for ending the day well.

So, these are some simple and effective 30 day meal plans for getting back in shape easily.

CHAPTER FOUR
30 DAY MEAL PREP TO GET IN SHAPE

The most effective way is typically to continually get back to the fundamentals as well as making use of what works. Stick to good information and you should not follow the newest diets or even fads on losing weight and you're going to be fine. Now we will look into how nutrition along with what you take in may help you lose a substantial amount of unwanted weight.

What to eat

Water rich food items

Try eating plenty of water rich foods which includes vegetables along with fruit. Water rich foods are not just beneficial, they can be a very important factor in shedding weight. Any of these water rich foods are actually very much less dense and don't deliver a great deal of calories but while doing so continue to keep us feeling satisfied. Water will also help to flush out impurities which happen to be one of several vehicles that stick in to additional fat in our body. The easiest way to make this happen should be to have a side salad with each and every meal that you have and additionally switch out snacks such as sugars to fruit.

Antioxidants and vitamin rich foods

Foods containing more antioxidants would be a requirement to include in your diet plan should you want to lose weight. Nearly all food items that are rich in antioxidants are great for slimming down as they are lower in calories. Vitamins also help our bodies perform better. With the body staying at a proper level, it is usually far easier to get rid of fat since the body stream is much smoother and takes away harmful toxins easier.

Things to refrain from

Unhealthy fats

What's as vital as picking the right foods is understanding what to steer clear of. This is an obvious one: refrain from fatty foods. This is really important simply because fatty foods don't just store as fat on your body but it makes you truly feel exhausted. Any time you feel really worn out you will find a higher chance you don't want to exercise as well. Unhealthy fats also block your system and therefore can make it more difficult for your body to cleanse and remove toxic compounds. These kinds of toxins keep hold of body fat and increases excess fat.

Sugar

Remember to keep far away from foods that have sugar. This includes candy, junk food, instant foods and more. Sugar is known as a supply of instant energy. The negative thing is if not burnt off, sugars can become extra fat and store in your body. Sugar is also high in calories and also low in nutrition. It is that which we call "empty calories". Foods which happen to be dense but are without any nutrients. Make sure you stick with purely natural sugars like fresh fruits rather than refined sugars which can do no good.

Since you now know exactly what to consume and just what not to consume, possibly the best way to lose more weight is generally to manage the portion you take in. Avoid overeating and you are on the right course. Even though it could be tough from time to time, the simplest way to accomplish this is to drink a big glass of water before you start to eat. This way, the body feels a bit more satiated just before you eat and it also helps clean out any toxic compounds which in turn helps to get rid of fat at the same time. A different way will be to save half your meal and eat it later. Eating a smaller amount but more often can help boost metabolism and this results in fat burning.

If you keep to the information above, you're going to be on the right track to creating your best physique. Reducing your weight isn't a difficult task and should not be overwhelming. Many weight loss trends help you to slim down but they do not keep us healthy and in most cases the excess weight returns. Maintaining everything we have discussed, it will be better to keep the body weight away once you get going and also stay in an improved condition. Therefore, begin your journey now and please remember the principles of a healthier lifestyle.

Would you believe it if someone told you that eating certain foods could help you lose unwanted pounds? Naturally you wouldn't, but it is true that certain foods can help in reducing your weight. Imagine losing weight simply because you eat more of these particular foods. Without a doubt, all these fat burning foods should be included in your diet. If you eat these foods three times a day, and remain active; you will be amazed at the results.

1. Beans: These contain a ton of protein, carbs, and fiber. They give you the fuel that your body needs to work, not feel hungry, and ensure that your body is working like it should. As a result, it's important to add beans to your dietary plan.

2. Cinnamon: Research indicates that consuming as little as a quarter tablespoon of cinnamon will maintain healthy blood sugar levels and increase insulin production. You'll have more energy while craving less sweets. In the end you won't be burdened with extra pounds.

3. Fish: Fish reduces leptin, a fatty acid which is needed. Leptin will offset obesity and the slowing down of your metabolism. Also, eating fish increases levels of omega-3 acids, which can be instrumental in keeping your heart in good shape. Therefore, fish is great to include in your diet as a way to stay healthy and lose weight.

4   Berries and Apples: Certain fruits such as berries and apples contain the water-binding ingredient pectin. Eating fruits that contain a lot

of pectin inhibits the absorption of fat and cholesterol. Therefore keeping unwanted fat away will be a lot easier.

5. Garlic may smell funny but it's a star in boosting metabolism and aiding weight loss.

6. Ginger: Ginger is a vasodilator, meaning that it expands the body's blood vessels. This raises the body's metabolic level, aiding in weight loss.

7. Soybeans: These beans can be a fantastic way to consume protein that is low in fat. Amazingly, it maintains a low glycemic index and a stable sugar level, so you can eat sweet foods with no effects.

8. Green tea: Great tea is better for you than coffee. It can increase your metabolism from 28% to 77% while at the same time refreshing you. The greater amount you consume, the more of an effect you will observe in the rate of your metabolism.

Lose 20 lbs In Two Weeks

In 1995, WHO (World Health Organisation) estimated that 200 million adults and 18 million children under 5 years of age are obese. In 2000, it reported that this figure has increased to more than 300 million. Hectic lifestyles is the most blamed factor. Overweight people are much prone to heart diseases, high blood pressure, cholesterol levels, hypertension, cancer, arthritis, sleep apnea, strokes, brain damage and diabetes. Apart from this, obese people also develop low self-esteem and have appearance issues. They are looked upon as unhappy, unhealthy, tired, sick or lazy individuals. Losing weight increases self-esteem, induces the feel good factor and enhances the appearance, besides preventing major diseases.

Therefore weight loss and fitness are issues of growing concern. People worldwide crave to shed their extra pounds and stay fit. Here we share with you some knowledge on how to lose 20 lbs in just two weeks. Of course, it takes a little bit effort on your part.

Dieting and exercising

Plan your diet. Say a big no to junk foods and carbonated drinks. Avoid all calorie rich foods.

Calculate your calorie intake, and restrict it to a certain level depending upon your energy requirements. Each and every single calorie counts when you are dieting.

Increase your metabolic rate, which is the rate at which your body processes and uses the food you eat. It is an easy and sensible technique to lose weight. Try taking several small meals a day instead of taking it in large amounts a few times a day. This burns your fats faster. Constant eating helps develop a higher metabolism within you in order to accommodate your frequent eating, hence burning calories fast.

Increase your physical activities, stay active, and include fibre rich diets to increase your metabolic rate. Including green tea in your daily fluid intake also helps in increasing your metabolism and energy level.

Go in for a detoxification of your system. It removes all the potentially harmful and toxic substances from your system and cleanses it. Follow a detox diet. Juice based detox diets are good options, especially, the lemonade diet. Detoxification helps you drop your liquid weight in a little time. Maintain a healthy lifestyle after detoxification.

Take eight glasses of water daily. Water plays an important role in weight loss by speeding up your metabolism and by ensuring proper digestion, besides rehydrating your body. Staying hydrated makes you feel more energetic, thus boosting your metabolic rate. Drinking water also reduces your strong craving for food.

Also, be sure to maintain your body's nutrition while dieting. Consume nutritious but low calorie food stuff. It is recommended that you cut 150-300 calories from your daily diet, and burn 150-300 calories in exercising. Scientific studies say, dieting is the best method for weight loss. But in order to achieve effective weight loss, doing a combo of dieting and exercising is necessary.

You will have to spend an hour or more to achieve your desired goal of losing 20 lbs in 2 weeks. Exercising should be intensive and vigorous, instead of merely walking. Doing the same kind of work outs render it boring. To ensure that it is interesting, do a variety of activities like jogging, cycling, weight lifting, hiking, rowing, etc. Doing some abdominal crunches keeps in check the belly contours. Exercises, besides giving your desired weight loss, also ensure that you are in a good shape. It does more good too.

Have the right mind set

To get motivated and to stay motivated are two important facets of your mind settings that will help you in reaching your predetermined goal of getting rid of those 20 lbs.

"Many of life's failures are people who did not realize how close they were to success when they gave up" - Thomas Edison.

Motivation and perseverance are essentials that keep you in the right mind set to help you attain your dream come true body weight. Motivation is the conscious or subconscious driving force, which when combines with steady persistence makes you achieve your goal. It contributes to your thoughts and actions.

Reason away: Why do you want to lose weight? Is it to look better? To feel more confident? To walk that ramp? To get that attention from your crush? Or anything else? You state it. Reasoning helps you take the necessary action by fixing your attitude.

Here are some points that will help you stay motivated:

- Make up your mind that you will never quit.

- Stay focussed on the end result.

- Keep track of your successes.

- Keep your motivation on high levels.

The thing next in getting the right mind set is positive thinking. There is a dramatic power in positive thinking. Positive thinking is a mental attitude that anticipates and admits conducive conditions in all the spheres of life in terms of growth, expansion and success. It is expressed through one's words and actions.

CHAPTER FIVE
THE PRONS AND CONS
OF LOW CARB DIET

Low carb diets are all the rage. They seem to work for many people, and these people swear by them. Unfortunately, they don't work for everyone who tries them. These people end up using an alternative method of weight loss. A low carbohydrate diet is basically cutting back or eliminating any foods which contain starches and carbohydrates and instead eating foods high in protein. For those who are curious about a low carb diet, you need to make sure it's right for you, your current health status, personal habits and lifestyle, and your ultimate goals.

With trying anything new, there are pros and cons to consider. And when it comes to dieting, you must be aware of all the issues related to your weight-loss and any weight-loss diet. The following gives you the "skinny" on the pros and cons in regards to low carbohydrate diets:

Pro - Because a low carbohydrate diet is all about eliminating carbs and not actual food, you can usually eat to your heart's content.

Con - Because you have to restrict yourself to certain foods, it can get monotonous.

Pro - Since low carb diets are so popular, you can find information about them quickly and easily.

Con - There is so much information about low carb diets it can get confusing and you still may not know everything you need to know before starting a low carb diet.

Pro - By eliminating foods high in carbs, you lose weight more quickly.

Con - When you eliminate certain food types, you also eliminate certain nutrients your body needs for optimal health.

Pro - It's easy to follow a low carb diet, the variety of foods can keep you satisfied.

Con - The foods you need to eat on a low carbohydrate diet can get expensive.

Pro - Low carb diets will get your cravings under control.

Con - You will go through withdrawals eating no or low carb foods only.

Pro - You will see faster weight loss when you eat low to no carbohydrate foods all the time.

Con - Low carb diets are harder to follow during special events, holidays and occasions when there are only high carb foods available.

Pro - Low carb diet are very effective for weight loss.

Con - To succeed on a low carbohydrate diet, you must have strong willpower.

Pro - Your immune system will improve with a low carbohydrate diet.

Con - Too many saturated fats are bad for the health of your heart.

Pro - You learn to eat healthier by ridding your body of carbs.

Con - Some carbs are not bad – complex carbs have nutritional value.

Pro - You will get high amounts of protein and can still enjoy eating the meats you love.

Con - People who are vegetarian will have trouble getting all the nutrition they need since they don't eat meat.

THE BASIC PRINCIPLE OF KETOGENIC DIET

One very popular weight loss program that many people are trying out are low carb diets. But, are low carb diets really that effective?

To an extent, yes, low carb diets can make dieting a great deal easier. Typically people using a low carb approach tend to have less hunger issues to deal with, tend to see reduced bloating, hence they look thinner, and also tend to enjoy the food since you're allowed to have more dietary fat with these approaches.

But, that said, there are some important things you must realize before starting up on a low carb diet. If you don't recognize these factors, you could wind up getting into quite a bit of trouble on a low carb diet and not see the types of results you're looking for.

Here's what you need to know about low carb diets.

Low Carb Diets And Exercise Carbs

First, it's going to be very important that you are having carb ups at some point during your exercise workout. This can be before or after the workout is finished, or in the form of one very large carb-up on the weekend. Doing so will help to ensure that the body has enough muscle glycogen storage to be able to continue on with the exercise programs you are asking it to perform.

Neglecting to take in carbs at this point can lead to feelings of fatigue, and may even cause you to stop your fat loss workouts altogether.

Low Carb Diets Shouldn't Limit Vegetables

Next, you also want to be sure you're not limiting vegetables at all while on a low carb diet. Doing so would be very problematic because these are filled with plenty of vitamins, minerals, and antioxidants.

Not too mention they are low in calories, high in fiber, and are one of the best diet foods to be eating.

So, don't limit your vegetable consumption even if you are on a low carb diet. You will want to watch out for the varieties that do contain more starch, such as peas, corn, and carrots, but otherwise you can eat quite a few without worry.

Low Carb Diets and Water Intake

Finally, the last thing to keep in mind is that low carb diets do tend to have a dehydrating effect on the body, therefore it's going to be very important that you make sure you're drinking plenty of liquids.

It would be a smart move to bump up your water intake slightly from what you'd normally drink – about 10-12 cups of fluid altogether should be plenty.

So, be sure you're keeping these points in mind when considering a low carb approach. While some people just do not feel well at all on low-carb diets, many others do have good success on them.

CHAPTER SIX
WHAT IS THE KETO DIET?

The keto diet involves going long spells on extremely low (no higher than 30g per day) to almost zero g per day of carbs and increasing your fats to a really high level (to the point where they may make up as much as 65% of your daily macronutrients intake.) The idea behind this is to get your body into a state of ketosis. In this state of ketosis the body is supposed to be more inclined to use fat for energy, and research says it does just this. Depleting your carbohydrate/glycogen liver stores and then moving onto fat for fuel means you should end up shredded.

You then follow this basic platform from say Monday until Sat 12pm (afternoon) (or Sat 7pm, depending on whose version you read). Then from this time until 12 midnight Sunday night (so up to 36 hours later) you carb up.

(Some say, and this will also be dictated by your body type, that you can go nuts in the carb up and eat anything you want and then there are those that more wisely – in my view – prescribe still sticking to the clean carbs even during your carb up.)

So calculating your numbers is as simple as the following...

Calculate your required maintenance level of daily calories...

(if you are looking to drop quickly use 1300. I would not advise this, if you want a more level drop in body fat use 1500 and if you are going to actually attempt to maintain or possibly put on some lean muscle mass then use 1700)

Body weight in pounds x 15= a

Protein for the day 1g per body weight in pounds= b

Bx4=c (c= number of calories allotted to your daily protein allowance).

a-c= d (d= amount of calories to be allotted to fat intake).

D/9= g per day of fat to be consumed.

The end calculation should leave you with a very high number for your fat intake.

Now for those of you wondering about energy levels: Especially for training because there are no carbs, with there being such a high amount of fat in the diet you feel quite full and the fat is a very good fuel source for your body. One adaptation that I have made is to actually have a nice fish fillet about an hour before I train and I find it gives me enough energy to get through my workout. (I am aware of the arguments made to not have fats 2-3 hours either side of training. While I won't have fats 2-3 hours after training as I want quick absorption and blood flow, I see no issue with slowing everything down before training so my body has access to a slow digesting energy source).

There are some that say to have a 30g carb intake immediately after training – just enough to fill liver glycogen levels. And then there are those that say having even as much as that may push you out of ketosis, the state you are trying to maintain.

During my carb up period, for the sake of those who would like to know if you can get in shape and still eat the things you want (in moderation), for the first six weeks I will be relaxed about what I eat in this period but then the following 6 weeks I will only eat clean carbs.

I also like to make sure that the first workout of the week — as in a Monday morning workout — is a nice long full hour of work so I start cutting into the liver glycogen immediately.

KETOGENIC DIETS AND WEIGHT LOSS AND BODYBUILDING

A ketogenic diet is one where there are no carbs. Without carbohydrates the body burns fat as the primary fuel source. Since this is happening the body can tap into stored bodyfat for energy and we can end up leaner. While that is possible we need to look at what may happen.

For starters your energy will be drained. Without carbohydrates your body won't know what energy source to turn to for a few days so you may experience feelings of weakness while you train or until your body becomes adapted to using fat. While this isn't a bad thing you must understand that you have to change your training intensity. There's no way that you can keep training at a high intensity while you use one of these diets.

The next thing that you have to understand about using a ketogenic diet for weight loss or bodybuilding is that you need to eat more protein then normal. Since you don't have carbs, and carbs are protein sparing, you need to consume more protein so you don't lose muscle tissue. So make sure that you are eating at least six meals per day with a serving of protein coming every meal.

Then you have to make sure that you are getting enough fiber. Look to consume fiber from various sources such as green vegetables and fiber powder or pills like physillum husk. Now you need to add some healthily nutritional supplements since you want to make sure that you do your best to burn fat on these keto diets for weight loss and bodybuilding. First, make sure you consume healthy fats like omega-3 fish oils, cla, and gla. These fats will help to burn more body fat. Then you want to purchase a good branch chain amino acid powder as bcaas help to retain muscle mass and prevent muscle breakdown.

KETOGENIC DIETS FOR MANAGING TYPE 2 DIABETES

Ketogenic diets have been in use since 1924 in pediatrics as a treatment for epilepsy. A ketogenic (keto) diet is one that is high in fat and low in carbs.

The design of the ketogenic diet is to shifts the body's metabolic fuel from burning carbohydrates to fats. With the keto diet, the body metabolizes fat, instead of sugar, into energy. Ketones are a byproduct of that process.

Over the years, ketogenic diets have been used to treat diabetes. One justification was that it treats diabetes at its root cause by lowering carbohydrate intake leading to lower blood sugar, which in turn, lowers the need for insulin which minimizes insulin resistance and associated metabolic syndrome. In this way, a ketogenic diet may improve blood glucose (sugar) levels while at the same time reducing the need for insulin. This point of view presents keto diets as a much safer and more effective plan than injecting insulin to counteract the consumption of high carbohydrate foods.

A keto diet is actually a very restrictive diet. In the classic keto diet for example, one gets about 80 percent of caloric requirements from fat and 20 percent from proteins and carbohydrates. This is a marked departure from the norm where the body runs on energy from sugar derived from carbohydrate digestion but by severely limiting carbohydrates, the body is forced to use fat instead.

A ketogenic diet requires healthy food intake from beneficial fats, such as coconut oil, grass-pastured butter, organic pastured eggs, avocado, fish such as salmon, cottage cheese, avocado, almond butter and raw nuts (raw pecans and macadamia). People on ketogenic diets avoid all bread, rice, potatoes, pasta, flour, starchy vegetables, and most dairy. The diet is low in vitamins, minerals, and nutrients and requires supplementation.

A low carbohydrate diet is frequently recommended for people with type 2 diabetes because carbohydrates turn to blood sugar which in large quantities cause blood sugar to spike. Thus, for a diabetic who already has high blood sugar, eating additional sugar-producing foods is like courting danger. By switching the focus from sugar to fat, some patients can experience reduced blood sugar.

Changing the body's primary energy source from carbohydrates to fat leaves behind the byproduct of fat metabolism, ketones in the blood. For some diabetic patients, this can be dangerous as a buildup of ketones may create a risk for developing diabetic ketoacidosis (DKA). DKA is a medical emergency requiring immediate medical attention. DKA signs include consistently high blood sugar, dry mouth, polyuria, nausea, breath that has a fruit-like odor and breathing difficulties. Complications can lead to a diabetic coma.

For many people, the ketogenic diet is a great option for weight loss. It is very different and allows the person on the diet to eat a diet that consists of foods that you may not expect.

When you eat a very low amount of carbs your body gets put into a state of ketosis. What this means is your body burns fat for energy. How low of an amount of carbs do you need to eat in order to get into ketosis? Well, it varies from person to person, but it is a safe bet to stay under 25g net carbs. Many would suggest that when you are in the "induction phase" which is when you are actually putting your body into ketosis, you should stay under 10g net carbs.

If you aren't sure what net carbs are, let me help you. Net carbs are the amount of carbs you eat minus the amount of dietary fiber. So if on the day you eat a total of 35g of net carbs and 13g of dietary fiber, your net carbs for the day would be 22. Simple enough, right?

So besides weight loss what else is good about keto? Well, many people talk about their improved mental clarity when on the diet. Another benefit is having an increase in energy. Yet another is a decreased appetite.

One thing to worry about when going on the ketogenic diet is something called "keto flu." Not everyone experiences this, but for those that do it can be tough. You will feel lethargic and you may have a headache. It won't last very long. When you feel this way make sure you get plenty of water and rest to get through it.

If this sounds like the kind of diet you would be interested in, then what are you waiting for? Dive head first into keto. You won't believe the results you get in such a short amount of time.

CHAPTER SEVEN
HOW TO ENSURE YOUR VEGAN MEALS AND RECIPES ARE LOW-CALORIE

Vegan Weight Loss Advice

Certain folk have trouble losing weight on the vegan lifestyle. Although the majority will experience weight loss on the vegan diet, there are always some who wonder what they are doing wrong. There are simple and easy measures that you can take to ensure that all of your vegan meals and recipes that you prepare are complementing your weight loss efforts.

1. Go steady with the oil

Olive oil and other healthy oils are essential for optimal health and will help keep your hair, skin and nails beautiful. However, because olive oil is a form of fat (the healthy type), it is very high in energy content. Therefore, to keep your vegan meals low-calorie you should measure out your olive oil with a spoon just as your recipes call for, rather than simply pouring the oil into your dish.

2. Keep an eye on your nut portions

Many vegan recipes feature walnuts, brazil nuts or other gourmet nuts to make the meal flavoursome and satisfying. If you are hoping to see some weight loss, however, only add nuts to one of your meals per day – not all three! This will help keep your diet low-calorie and low-fat and will ultimately result in a slimmer physique.

3. Don't eat too much vegan junk-food

You should endeavour to make your own wholesome vegan meals and recipes as often as you are able, rather than opting for quick vegan junk food. This will make you in control of your food, and you can make your vegan meals and recipes as low-calorie and low-fat as you please. Vegan junk food on the other hand is terrible for weight loss, with packet chips, cookies, chocolates, salty nuts and soft-drinks the main offenders. These foods are too high in energy to eat on a regular basis, so please stick to making your own fresh vegan meals to guarantee weight loss.

4. Share your vegan baking with your friends

There are so many beautiful and tasty vegan sweets and dessert recipes that you can make nowadays, and let's be fair, every vegan should enjoy their fair share. But when you do bake, only make one serving of the recipe rather than doubling or tripling it. Also, share your recipes with friends, family and colleagues to show a giving spirit and mostly to save yourself from unnecessary emotional eating.

You can take control of your calorie intake on the vegan diet to ensure a steady weight loss. Remember to go steady with the olive oil, keep an eye on you nut portions, limit your vegan junk-food and share your baking with friends. Making wise choices as such will help make your weight loss a sure success on the vegan diet.

VEGAN MEAL PLAN

Switching to a vegan diet can be a great way to lose weight and get healthier. A vegan does not eat any foods that contain or are made with animal products of any kind. This can be a restrictive lifestyle, but many people choose to make this change and it is no surprise with all the weight that can be lost. No matter if it is due to religious reasons, health reasons, or concern for animal welfare, a vegan diet can really change how you feel and how you look.

If you are thinking about making the move to a vegan lifestyle it might help for you to have a vegan meal plan. There are so many delicious options for vegan foods. This meal plan is just a jumping off point. It is a great idea to buy some vegan cookbooks. It is also great to check out the thousands of vegan recipes that are online. Be adventurous and try new things. Here are some vegan recipes for breakfast, lunch, dinner, and dessert.

Breakfast

- Scrambled Tofu
- 1 ½ tablespoon safflower oil
- 3 tablespoons diced onion
- 1 diced Serrano chili
- 1/2 teaspoon ground cumin
- 3 tablespoons chopped cilantro
- 20 oz tofu
- Salsa of your choosing

Instructions

Heat the oil; add in onion and sauté for 1 to 2 minutes. Add the chilies and cumin, cook for a few minutes. Crumble the tofu and cook, stirring frequently. Mix in the cilantro and season with salt. Serve with warm tortillas and salsa.

Lunch

- Sweet Corn Soup
- 6 ears of corn
- 1 tablespoon corn oil
- 1 small onion
- 1/2 cup grated celery root
- 7 cups water or vegetable stock
- Salt to taste

1. Shuck the corn and slice off the kernels.

2. In a large soup pot put in the oil, onion, celery root, and one cup of water. Let that mixture stew under low heat until the onion is soft.

3. Add the corn, salt and remaining water and bring it to a boil.

4. Cool briefly and then puree in a blender, then wait for it to cool before putting it through a food mill.

5. Reheat and add salt and pepper to taste.

Dinner

Seared Portobello Mushrooms

- 1 large Portobello mushroom, stem removed
- Olive oil as needed
- Salt and pepper
- Shallot vinaigrette

1. Slice the mushroom into wide slices.

2. Brush both sides with oil and set them in the skillet over high heat. Sear for 4 to 5 minutes.

3. Once they start to brown remove them and place them on a platter with salt and pepper to taste.

4. Add vinaigrette to the top for flavor.

Lentil and Onion Croquettes

- 2 cups chopped yellow onion
- 2 tablespoons olive oil
- 1/2 cup finely chopped carrot
- 2 cups bread crumbs
- 1 cup lentils
- 3/4 cup celery chopped
- Salt and pepper

1. In a skillet over low heat cook the onion in the olive oil.

2. In a saucepan combine the lentils, celery, carrots, and salt covered with water. Bring this to a boil and then lower the heat to a simmer for about 30 minutes.

3. Drain the liquid. Puree the lentils until smooth.

4. Mix the lentils with the onion and bread crumbs. Season with salt and pepper.

5. Allow the mixture to cool and then form it into 3 inch rounds. Fry the croquette balls in olive oil and set them on a paper towel to soak up the excess oil.

Dessert

Strawberry Ice

- 1 quart ripe strawberries
- Stevia (to taste)

1. Pull out the core of the berries.

2. Puree them in a food processor.

3. Put stevia into a saucepan. Add half a cup of the puree into the stevia and heat stirring constantly until it is all dissolved.

4. Add in the puree and freeze.

CHAPTER EIGHT
STAYING HEALTHY WITH VEGAN MEALS ON A KETO DIET

There are many reasons why people should be careful with what they eat. First off, they have too many activities to attend to every day. With each activity, their body consumes and burn energy. The environment is also no longer as safe as it was. Even the air that supplies the oxygen contains particles and bacteria that could cause diseases. One way to protect their body from diseases is by eating healthy and nutritious food.

Nowadays, people try to keep their bodies protected and healthy through exercise and healthy diets. Many people follow a vegetarian diet plan. However, even with this plan, people may still be at risk of some illnesses.

When a person prepares a meal, he has to remember that every ingredient he uses is special and is meant for something. Some ingredients are used to give the meal a pleasing taste. But, most ingredients are used to infuse it with nutrients and vitamins that the body needs.

Meat, for example, is a good source of protein. Proteins act as the building blocks of the body. They are needed to develop the muscles, cartilages, and bones. Even skin and blood needs them. Without them, you may stay in the gym the whole day and obtain very little result. Going for high protein, low carb vegetarian foods is actually going to help you have stronger muscles and a leaner body.

Carbohydrate is another component that the human body needs. It is what keeps people doing what they have to do by helping them obtain energy. Unfortunately, having too much of it could lead to serious and long-term diseases like diabetes and high blood pressure. In fact, dieticians and other health experts recommend some low carb vegetarian recipes to people suffering from such conditions.

People who try to indulge in vegetarian meals without understanding how it works may deny their body some nutrients. That is because this diet may not include the sources of proteins, carbohydrates and some vitamins that are required by the body.

On the other hand, following a vegan meal may actually be a good start to a healthier lifestyle. But, a person who intends to shift to this kind of diet should first look at what he needs. He must consider his activities and health conditions. He needs to determine what he actually wants to develop or remove from his body. Taking these things into consideration would help him obtain faster results, and a fitter and healthier body. Most importantly, it would help him determine what vegetarian diet plan to follow.

On the vegan diet you should experience a profound detoxification of your body, a restoral of your health, a newfound zest for life, and of course, weight loss. Most folk who go on the vegan diet will lose weight, but there are the minority who do not. What are they doing wrong? Let's look at several mistakes that they may be making which are greatly sabotaging their weight loss efforts.

1. Over-eating

All foods should be eaten in moderation – regardless of how healthy they are. For example, one single banana is low in calories (approximately 100). Most vegans love bananas and will happily consume two or three a day. But what if you had 10 bananas in one day plus your other meals? This means that you will be consuming 1000 calories per day with bananas alone. This may sound like a crazy example, but I'm sure it gets the point across. You should eat all foods in moderation. Eat generous sized meals but don't make yourself sick. Eat your meals with intuition, balance and self-control. This will ensure that you will lose weight on the vegan diet.

2. Too many Nuts

Nuts are an essential food for those on the vegan diet due to their high nutritional properties, particularly for their protein and healthy-fat content. But the problem is when you have too many as the calories add up fast. Many folk say that they can easily polish off an entire container of nuts in one sitting. I'm sorry to say this, but if you intend to lose weight on the vegan diet, you need to limit your serving of nuts. Don't deprive yourself of them, but one or two handfuls per day should be sufficient.

3. Too much oil

Olive oil and other healthy oils are very good for your hair, skin and nails and you should consume a couple of tablespoons every day. But these oils are also very high in calorie content so please measure out your servings with a spoon, rather than happily pour the oil into your dish like a free-spirited chef. Just remember, by sensibly measuring out your olive oil you can keep your vegan meals low-calorie and low-fat. This will in turn help you to lose weight.

4. Too many avocadoes

Avocadoes are considered one of the top superfoods in the world. Due to their super-high nutrient content, they can help boost your health and make you beautiful on the inside and outside. But they are also high in energy due to their healthy fat content, so please stick to half to one medium sized avocado per day. Limiting your avocado portions will help ensure that your vegan meals will be low-fat and low-calorie.

5. Vegan Junk-Food

Nobody should eat much junk food, whether vegan or not. The vegan junk food list is long, with the common rogues being packet chips, biscuits, chocolate, lollies and soft-drinks. So stay away from these foods most of the time and only have these on special occasions. It's all about eating in moderation. Eat this food only a couple of times per week rather than on a daily basis.

These are the most common causes why some vegans cannot lose weight. Really, the key is to enjoy your vegan food in moderation, limit your portion of nuts, oils and avocadoes, and steer away from vegan junk food.

Benefits of a Vegan Lifestyle

One common notion about becoming a vegan is that you'll miss foods that are not part of the diet, such as meat. However, most people who begin following a plant-based diet come to find it expansive and empowering instead of restrictive. The truth is you will eat better than you did in the past and feel better as well. Cravings for meat, fish, and dairy products will dissipate over time until they are not missed. If you are thinking about becoming a vegan, below are six benefits of the lifestyle that may help your decision.

Deeper Compassion

A vegan's compassion extends its reach to all living creatures. With increased compassion comes greater acceptance of all life and the appreciation that it adds value to our own, making us stronger.

Expanded Palate

Vegans learn to enjoy a very wide range of vegetables which leads to an expanded palate. Recipes abound for cooking every vegetable imaginable. When veggies are just a side dish, it's convenient to settle for a few of them to complement meat, such as potato salad, peas and carrots, or corn. Once veggies are the main dish, however, one starts to appreciate many more ingredients enriching the dining experience.

Global Impact

The vegan lifestyle is much more than food. It's about the environment, climate, sustainable development, efficient allocation of food sources, and animal welfare. Many of the themes associated with going green are linked to veganism. When one chooses to be a vegan, one participates and supports these themes. The impact of eating vegan is so powerful, that if everyone did it constantly or even occasionally, many of these issues would resolve themselves.

Increased Mobility

Nutritionists, dietitians, and health scientists are confirming the health benefits of a plant-based diet over a meat-based one. Lower blood pressure, reduced risk of heart disease and cancer, and longer life spans are possible outcomes of a vegan diet. Fewer health problems mean that one is more active and mobile and can enjoy life more fully.

Larger Social Network

The vegan community is large and growing. Vegans enjoy sharing their experiences and finding companions who understand the reasons for their eating habits. Meeting and connecting with new people is one of the fun social aspects of being vegan.

New Knowledge

The vegan diet is focused on ingredients, health, and nutrition. To enjoy vegan food and stay healthy, one inevitably learns more about nutrition and the impact of ingredients on health. Over time, by paying attention to what it consumed and the value of each ingredient, one becomes familiar with vitamins, minerals, protein, fiber, antioxidants, and phytonutrients and with it comes new knowledge and power.

The benefits of a vegan lifestyle make one a more empowered person. New experiences lead to new ideas and new ways to enjoy and fully appreciate life. Try eating more vegan meals and enjoy the positive impact.

CHAPTER NINE
HOW TO FOLLOW A PLANT-BASED KETOGENIC DIET

So how exactly do you slip into ketosis without loading up on butter and bacon? And how can you ensure that your nutrient needs are still being met while following a plant-based ketogenic diet?

The key is to swap out your starchy veggies for low-carb alternatives while also filling your diet with plenty of plant-based fats and proteins. This can help you stay under your carbohydrate goal and provide your body with the important vitamins and minerals that it needs to stay healthy.

High-carb foods that should be limited in your diet include:

- High-Sugar Fruits (apples, oranges, bananas, grapes, etc.)

- Starchy vegetables (potatoes, sweet potatoes, winter squash, peas, corn, etc.)

- Sugar (including honey, maple syrup, agave syrup, etc.)

- Legumes (beans, lentils, peas, etc.)

- Grains (wheat products, rice, quinoa, cereal, etc.)

Instead, be sure to include plenty of nutrient-rich, low-carb plant-based foods in your diet, such as:

- Fermented foods (tempeh, natto, etc.)

- Leafy greens (kale, chard, spinach, collard greens, etc.)

- Non-starchy vegetables (asparagus, carrots, cauliflower, onions, mushrooms, peppers, etc.)

- Nuts (almonds, walnuts, pistachios, pecans, etc.)

- Seeds (chia seeds, flax seeds, hemp seeds, pumpkin seeds, etc.)

- Low-sugar fruits (blackberries, raspberries, strawberries, etc.)

- Healthy fats (coconut oil, MCT oil, olive oil)

Including enough protein in your diet can be challenging on any plant-based diet, let alone a plant-based ketogenic diet. Fortunately, there are tons of healthy options that can provide the protein you need to keep you going.

A few examples of low-carb, plant-based proteins include:

- Tempeh
- Natto
- Nutritional Yeast
- Spirulina
- Nuts
- Seeds

High-quality, low-sugar plant-based protein powders

Similarly, nixing all dairy products from your diet can make it tricky to get in enough fat, but there are plenty of plant-based sources of fat available that can help you easily meet your needs.

Some of the healthiest plant-based fats include:

- Avocado Oil
- Coconut Oil

- Olive Oil
- MCT Oil
- Avocado
- Nuts
- Seeds

Note that you can easily swap these nutritious foods into your favorite recipes to make them completely plant-based and keto-friendly. Nutritional yeast, for example, makes a great substitute for cheese while tempeh can be crumbled and cooked like ground beef to make delicious veggie tacos or lettuce wraps.

Sample Meal Plan:

Wondering what exactly a plant-based ketogenic diet looks like? Here's a one-day sample meal plan that you can follow to help get you started!

Breakfast:

Gluten-free oatmeal (2 grams net carbs per serving)

Lunch:

Baked tempeh (3 grams net carbs per serving)

Cauliflower tabbouleh salad (6 grams net carbs per serving)

Olive oil vinaigrette (0 grams net carbs per serving)

Dinner:

Raw walnut tacos (4 grams net carbs per serving)

Super cilantro guacamole (5 grams net carbs per serving)

Snacks:

Keto smoothie with avocado, chia seeds & cacao (6.5 grams net carbs)

Almonds (2.5 grams net carbs per 1-oz serving)

Spicy roasted pumpkin seeds (10 grams carbs per 1-oz serving)

Daily Total: 39 grams net carbs

WHAT VEGASs EAT IN THEIR KETO JOURNEY

But can a vegetarian or vegan be Keto? Does the necessity of fat and the small margin for carbs eliminate anyone else except meat and dairy consumers? No. The vegetarian and vegan can still be LCHF while observing their food preferences. Here at Keys to Ketosis, we've provided a vegan ketogenic diet food list to help anyone who is conscious of what types of food they consume, but still wants to (or has to) pursue a low-carb, high-fat lifestyle.

Check out the list of compiled low-carb vegan diet below!

Tofu

The point of tension for a vegan/vegetarian attempting to pursue a LCHF will be the choices for a base food or "main course" food that will provide much of their protein and fat sources.

On the vegan ketogenic diet food list, tofu will be one of the big operators for finding interesting ways to creating mindful food that also assists you in your low-carb pursuit. Tofu is a versatile food, that comes in various forms and can be cooked in a variety of ways, including grilling, frying, baking, or just eating it raw. Having this on your vegan ketogenic diet food list will be imperative to maintaining excitement and variety.

Tofu Nutriton Facts (1/2 Cup):

Calories: 94

Fats: 6g

Carbs: 2.3g

Protein: 10g

Nuts

Nuts are a must on the Ketogenic diet, but peanuts should be eaten judiciously, due to their classification of legume, which means they belong to the same family as beans, and share their high carb profiles. However, you can use peanut butter for a topping, but once again, not in excess.

The good news for your vegan ketogenic diet food list is that there are plenty of nuts that are permissible – and beneficial – to being low-carb high-fat.

The best of the best include the following (in descending order from best to worst):

- Almonds
- Macadamia Nuts
- Walnuts
- Pecans
- Cashews and Pistachios

Nut based flours can also be used for baking instead of high-carb wheat flour.

MCT Oil

MCT Oil will make staying LCHF on a vegan diet easier than it has ever been.

MCT oil for keto diet plan

By using this supplement in shakes, as a dressing, or on other foods, you can ensure that your body is getting the correct doses of fatty acids that are essential to ketosis.

Other ideas:

Mixing in toppings (like mayo)

Use while baking food instead of regular baking oil

The great thing about using MCT Oil (and other exogenous ketones) is that you can counterbalance some of the carbs you will inevitably take by adhering to the vegan ketogenic diet food list.

Olive and Coconut Oil

Other oils that are great for toppings or cooking are coconut and olive oil. Both of these oils provide a great source of healthy fats, and a broad range of uses for food.

And unlike MCT Oil, these oils can be used for frying and sautéing food. Coconut oil is more stable than olive oil, so it is the better choice for using at high temperatures.

The benefit that these two oils bring to your vegan ketogenic diet food list, is their ability to provide vibrancy with flavor. While MCT Oil can provide a more potent shot of healthy fat, it can also bring with it a taste that can be hard to handle if not masked, whereas coconut and olive oil are both pleasurable to consume.

Greens

Since fruits are a no-no on the ketogenic diet (except for avocados), you will need to be strategic about eating enough greens to get the nutrients you'd get from the fruits you'd normally consume on a standard vegan diet.

The vegetables that you should keep stocked on your ketogenic diet food list are leafy greens like kale, collard greens, spinach, swiss chard, and others of the same family.

These vegetables, mixed with avocados and keto friendly oils (listed above) will help you stay vibrant from proper vitamin intake, while also helping you maintain a low-carb lifestyle.

Fatty Produce (Avocado)

The avocado is the hallmark of healthy fats from fruits (yes, avocados are a fruit). It is also capable of being used in every meal of the day, pairing well with salads. Did we mention that guacamole is incredible?

Avocados are considered a superfood, because of the research that suggests they help lower cholesterol, and even ward off cancer!

Nutrition Info (1 avocado):

Calories: 322
Fats: 29g
Carbs: 17g
Protein: 4g

CONCLUSION

What does it mean to be on a keto meal (often shortened to "keto") diet? When you're on a keto diet, you consume a very low-carb, high-fat diet. The idea behind this way of eating and why it can work so well is that when the body gets such small amounts of glucose from carbohydrates, it can burn another fuel source — fat — for energy. This is why the keto diet is known for helping the body to burn fat impressively fast! What if you're not trying to lower the number on your scale? The keto diet still may appeal to you since by limiting sugars and processed grains, you may lower your risk of developing type 2 diabetes, a disease which is becoming more and more common these days.

www.ingramcontent.com/pod-product-compliance
Lightning Source LLC
Chambersburg PA
CBHW071458030726
47593CB00003B/1049